Exercises for Noticing Mindfully Volume Three

Mindfulness Practices for Persons with Parkinson's Disease

9/3/2014
Parkinsons Recovery
Robert Rodgers PhD

Contents

The Parkinsons Recovery Mindfulness Series

Realistically speaking, how can the intense level of stress that aggravates the symptoms of Parkinson's disease be calmed? Better yet, how can they be quieted? My research over the past decade reveals that using your mind to drop the stress level down a notch or two always backfires. When you tell yourself:

- *Settle down!*
- *Take it easy!*
- *Stop being so stressed out!*

The stress level ratchets up, not down. Attempts to force the stress and anxiety levels to adjust downward induce an internally generated stress. They pile more stress on top of an excess of stress that already exists. There are certainly a sufficient number of external generators of stress in every one's life. Why infuse more stress that you create yourself, even with the best of intentions?

If the mind is not a useful technique to reduce stress, what is? The most eloquent answer I have for you is to become more mindful of what is experienced in the present moment. Becoming more mindful shifts you into the experience of the "now" which in itself is less stressful (unless you have been kidnapped by terrorists!).

It is stressful to anticipate events you imagine will occur in the future. The events we imagine rarely happen. Does this ring true for you? We all create unnecessary stress in our lives by how and where we focus our thoughts and attention.

It is stressful to agonize over the past. When we think about the past, we are much more likely to think about unpleasant experiences that induce stress. The past event itself was traumatic enough. Yet, we insist on reliving the trauma over and over again through our memories. It seems some of us just can't get enough stress in our lives.

The problem with upping the ante on stress levels is that – as you well know – symptoms of Parkinson's disease become worse. When you are not as stressed, your symptoms are far less problematic.

I have reached one solid conclusion from my ten years of research on Parkinson's disease. Symptoms will drive you crazy when you are stressed and are far less problematic when stress is under control.

Now, if you can't use your mind to become more mindful (which creates added stress in itself) how in the world can you quiet down a frantic lifestyle? I have concluded that the simplest and most effective solution to reducing stress levels is to become more mindful.

The transformation is possible step by step through these simple exercises you can do anywhere, anytime of the day. The Parkinsons Recovery mindfulness exercises are designed to focus your attention on the present moment as attention on either the past or the future is diverted. A renewed focus on the present moment reduces stress levels. Mindfulness is a lifestyle that will reduce stresses in your life if you set the intention to take a mindfulness practice seriously.

I recommend that you practice each of the exercises for a week or longer. Incorporate each practice into your regular routines and habits. Attempts to do all of the exercises simultaneously will likely induce more stress which – obviously – is contrary to the intent of a successful mindfulness program.

Give each exercise a little time and space. Invite the stresses in your life to dissipate. Allow the experience of each practice to engulf you. In so doing, watch the stresses in your life dip down to new lows along with a concurrent relief of any and all symptoms that you have currently been experiencing.

This volume is one out of nine that I have written to support the recovery of persons who currently experience neurological symptoms. A full listing of the Parkinsons Recovery Mindfulness themes follows:

Exercises for Noticing Mindfully
Mindfulness Practices for Persons with Parkinson's Disease
Volume Three

Robert Rodgers, PhD

Parkinsons Recovery

www.parkinsonsrecovery.me

Olympia, Washington

How Do You Define Your Territory?

My challenge for you this week is to become aware and mindful of how you define the territory that is yours and yours alone. More specifically, how do you label and define who you are? How do you assert and declare ownership of very specific places on this earth? The challenge of the week is not about being aware so you can stop labeling yourself or defining yourself. We all have labels. It is becoming mindful and aware of what labels we attach to ourselves and what territories we associate ourselves with. Some examples will help and by way of introduction.

Do you tend to think of yourself as a:

- **Conservative or Liberal?**
- **Democrat or Republican?**
- **East coast or a West coast or Midwest or Southwest person or none of these?**

When people ask, "*what do you do*" what is your answer?

- *Mother*
- *Housewife*
- *House husband*
- *Professor*
- *Politician*
- *Lawyer*

- *Artist*
- *Researcher*
- *Plumber*
- *Salesperson*

What do you say when asked, *"What do you do?"* Do you say

> *"I'm retired?"*

Do you say,

> *"I'm between jobs?"*

What is the label that you most closely associate with? How do you respond when you are ask this question? When people ask me this question I tend to slip myself into different categories depending on the situation. I think of myself as a researcher. I think of myself as a writer. I think of myself as a facilitator or mediator. There are many, many other labels that I identify with.

The second component of defining your territory and becoming mindful of how you stake out your territory is to become aware of those special places that you declare to be yours and yours alone. Perhaps:

- *A special chair that you and only you are allowed or invited to sit in.*
- *A desk that is yours, not a shared desk.*

7

- *A walking route that you take which is patently yours.*
- *A table at a restaurant-when you walk in you are bound and determined to wait for a very specific table because that happens to be your personal table.*
- *A lane on the expressway that is your lane and not to be shared with anyone else.*
- *A chair at your own dinner table or breakfast table.*

What is your territory and how do you define it?

In some ways I am inviting you this week to become a two-year-old who is very assertive and vocal about their territory. When certain toys are thought to be the two-year-old toys, they will very loudly and profusely declare, "Mine."

The invitation this week then is become aware of the territory that you declare for yourself. May you have a delightful time becoming aware of how you define your territory.

Deeper Meaning Behind Territorial Declarations

What is the deeper meaning behind a mindfulness challenge that asked you to become aware of the territories that you declare for yourself, the labels that you affix to who you are? Territories are fixed, immutable entities. They are declarations of how everything should be now. Territories that are here today, however, are oftentimes gone tomorrow.

The high school which I attended, Sandy Springs High School in Atlanta, Georgia, no longer exists. It was torn down and replaced by a Home Depot. The Navy base where I worked as a navy officer in Puerto Rico known as Roosevelt Roads has been sold to private developers. The graduate program I attended at Cornell University is no longer offered. It was a Masters of Public Administration in the business school. They decided that they would only offer a Masters of Business Administration rather than a Masters of Public Administration. Many of the publishers who have published my work no longer exist. They have gone out of business.

Here today. Gone tomorrow.

Our ideas are also territories in themselves. I have throughout my lifetime possessed many ideas that I was absolutely certain were correct; I knew my thinking was right and the thinking of others was wrong. I was willing

9

to do anything to assert the righteousness and correctness of my thoughts. Over time I have begun to recognize that many, many – and might I add one more, many – of these ideas have been actually dead wrong. My thinking was, I must confess—flawed. What I thought to be true and right as it turns out was just the opposite.

When we get upset about invasions of our territory, we often – and my hand is raised – get angry or irritated. When my territory is invaded, I feel my blood pressure rise. I have a chair which I declare to be my chair at the dinner table. When anyone else sits in it I can feel my blood pressure rise.

Might I now admit, isn't that reaction absolutely silly? Consider the many ways territories get invaded. A neighbor has a dog that barks late at night. The response is to think,

> *"Now, if my neighbor would just move, all of my problems would be solved."*

Of course we all know deep down inside that this hope is seldom delivered in reality. If the old neighbor does move for whatever reason, the new neighbor might not have any dogs whatsoever, or camels, or deer, but they may like to have parties that go on until two o'clock in the morning.

Are we going to spend our life hoping that someone will leave and die so that our lives will be made perfect? We may think to ourselves,

> *"I look 60."*

What a label for a person who is 40. That is a declaration that certainly is not in their best and highest good. The reality is that most of us are very ignorant about our true selves. The self is always changing. The body is always in flux. And yes – our age is always shifting.

Take an imaginary super-microscope and apply that microscope to any tissues on your body. You will see a living organism that has many, many living entities that are interacting, interfacing and communicating with one another. There are billions and billions of life forces contained within our body. Your body, my body is not the same now as it was when you began to read this section.

We are always in flux. We are always changing. A thought form that says ...

> *"If symptom X or symptom Y or symptom Z will just vanish I will be good to go."*

Is the same as imposing a territorial requirement on your body. Symptoms emerge. Symptoms vanish. Our bodies are in continuous flux. Our bodies do tend to push out of balance during one point of the day or another. There are

11

biorhythms that we must respect. There are cycles of sugar levels that are always moving upward and downward as a function of what we are ingesting.

The body may be able to suppress symptoms, but your kidneys, liver and heart will likely be compromised! That is certainly a side effect no one wishes to experience.

Reifying and concretizing a sense of self only creates anxiety, stress and suffering. Acknowledge and accept that your body is a miracle, always able to respond and adjust, though at times those responses and those adjustments may create pain, discomfort and emotional distress. Respect the self as a living, mutable, gorgeous entity that is changing moment by moment. Becoming mindful of the current situation (rather than labeling it) reduces anxiety, releases stress and ensures that symptoms are unable and unlikely to flare.

Enjoy the rest of the week as you become more and more mindful of all of the territories that you declare for yourself, of all the anger and irritation that arises when those territories are invaded. I say again, much of what I was certain is true turns out not to be true today.

I admit at this place and this time and this hour that much of what I think in this hour may also prove to be untrue and false.

- **May my thoughts be fluid.**

12

- **May they be agile.**
- **May I accept my body as a creative entity able to respond to whatever challenges it confronts.**

The mantra of the week is –

In this space of fluidity, of flexibility, of malleability, of openness to change, of being in the moment

I declare here and now to be in the present, celebrating all that the present entails.

Becoming mindful of the present moment is the gateway to true health and wellness.

13

Balance

The invitation this week is actually simple to do. Whenever you find you are standing anywhere; looking at flowers, standing while someone else talks with you or you talk with them, standing while you are waiting in line to purchase an item at the grocery store or hardware store – just standing – notice whether or not the weight is evenly distributed between your right foot and leg and your left foot and leg. Or, notice whether you are placing more weight and force on one leg than the other.

For example, are you literally lifting one leg up and placing the tips of the toes on the floor or the ground and forcing all of the weight onto either the right side or the left side? What is really happening when you stand? Notice.

It's a simple challenge. It is also a challenge that I have discovered has revealed incredible insights about the imbalances that I have created in my own body by way of habit. I, for one, have not been particularly mindful of how I was stressing certain muscles in my body unnecessarily when standing until I began to notice how I stood.

To summarize, each and every opportunity that you find yourself in a situation where you are standing – standing anywhere, standing for any reason – focus your attention on how much weight you are placing on each side of your body. If you notice that more weight is being placed on

14

either the left or the right foot and leg; redistribute the weight so that it is even across both sides of your body. Set the intention to stand firmly on Mother Earth.

Admittedly this is a simple challenge, but I must say for me personally it has had profound consequences for being able to balance out the stresses and strains that were exhibited throughout my body. We can do this moment by moment by being mindful.

I have an addendum to the exercise for this week. The addendum is notice how couples stand when they talk with one another a flirting way for perhaps the first time or a first date. I have noticed with great curiosity and interest how the man and how the woman stand when they talk with one another. It is generally a stressful context when a man is trying to impress the woman. Of course, the same observations may be seen when two men or two women who like each other are talking.

The question to ask is: How is each individual standing? Often I have noticed one of the people, if not both, are actually not standing on both feet; one of the feet is pitched upward rather than firmly planted on the ground. There is often great anxiety in such situations. The level of stress is off the charts. The stress and anxiety is evident from the observation that the individuals are not balanced and grounded and connected to Mother Earth.

Just notice as you look around, traveling from one place to another for the rest of the week, how people stand when they talk with one another. It is actually rare when you see two people who are firmly and evenly planted on the earth with energy that is evenly distributed between the right side and the left side.

Deeper Meaning Behind Balance

By way of explaining the deeper meaning behind the balance exercise I have a novel experience for you to consider right now. This experience is pure fantasy. It is not real, but one that I actually personally experienced when I attended my four-year healing school. It is an experience that gave me profound insights about my own body.

What I want to tell you at the outset is I am going to create a situation where in your imagination you are going to be frightened. Now know that this is not a real situation. There is absolutely no reason to be frightened. The entire idea is to fabricate a situation where you can experience what your body habitually does when you encounter something that is fearful. Once you imagine the situation I will ask you to freeze your body in that position so that you can sense which muscles you are tensing up and which side of your body is taking the brunt of the tension and the stress. Remember. This is an imagined situation that is supposed to frighten you. You are going to react with your

16

body and emotions. Then, you are going to freeze all of that for a few seconds.

Again (I hate to repeat myself but I was a professor for 20 years) this is not a real situation; it's just an exercise for you to experience what your body will feel like whenever you're under stress and whenever you are in fear (which for many people is several times a day). Here it goes.

> Imagine that you are having a wonderful day today. See yourself walking down a hiking path with gorgeous trees, with an individual by your side who you love dearly and who is your closest friend. You are talking with one another. You are having a grand time. You are taking sweet sips of water as you float down the trail. You stop for a few minutes to have a snack. It is a good day to be alive and it is a gorgeous hike.
>
> Suddenly, without notice, just 20 yards away, your walking partner notices a mama bear with two cub bears. Your partner says to you,
>
> > "Oh my God, it is a mama bear with her cubs. Look!"
>
> You look over, spot the bears and suddenly become frightened. Now, let your body be frightened right now. Just imagine you are actually looking at the

17

mama bear face to face. How are you reacting right now?

Where do your hands go? What about your body, your shoulders, your feet? Be shocked. Allow your body to react.

Now hold it. Freeze it. Freeze the shock right now. There is no need to hold the position for long - just a few seconds will do. Sense the tension is in your body. Where is it?

Notice. Be mindful. How is your body feeling now? Now, go ahead and relax.

This obviously didn't actually happen. Relax and now reflect on which muscles were tensing up when you became scared in that imaginary circumstance.

- *Was it your right side?*
- Was it your left side?
- *Was it your neck?*
- *Was it your shoulders?*
- *Was it your knee?*
- *Was it your calf muscles?*
- *Was it your stomach?*
- *Was it all of the above?*

What muscles did you tense up? Your body has reacted in the same fashion over and over and over again – every day, actually, although not to the extent that it will tense up when something truly fearful and scary happens like confronting a mother bear face to face.

The body becomes accustomed to using and stressing certain muscles. This stress creates a profound imbalance in the structure of the muscle interfaces. It becomes difficult to walk effortlessly. Balance becomes a problem because there is not an even distribution of how muscles are working in the left hand and right, in the left and right shoulders, the right and left legs, the right and left foot, etc.

When we are mindful of the extent to which we are stressing certain muscles of our body – wherever they might be located – much more frequently and much often than other muscles, we can redistribute that. Of course we need to be scared sometimes. Of course we need to tense up. We can't change that. But that very habit of reaction is going to create stresses and strains on the physical body that creates profound imbalances. This is the simple explanation for why so many people have back problems.

Reflexology is an emerging discipline which allows healing to occur by touching certain places on the feet. There is a connection to each and every organ, each and every blood vessel that is actually located somewhere on the toes, under the soles of the feet or on top of the feet. When confronting neurological challenges, many people tend to think over and over that the problem resides in the brain.

19

It is actually a full system issue. The key access point for healing is not in the brain. It is not through our thoughts. The door way actually opens up through our feet.

Randy Eady, better known as the Foot Whisperer, works with people who currently experience the symptoms of Parkinson's disease. Randy has shown why being more attentive to your feet does have profound implications for being able to reverse whatever symptoms you might be currently experiencing.

A final addendum to this week's challenge is to consider taking off your shoes on occasion, even your socks. Begin to walk around more often that way as you allow there to be a stimulation of the parts of your feet that may need to be stimulated. By stimulating all parts of the feet you are actually energizing and activating the lazy muscles and the all of the tired organs that may need a wake-up call.

Have fun as you notice the balance between the right and the left sides of your body. Feel free to imagine this week the experience of getting scared; perhaps as hiking as we just envisioned and encountering a mother bear with her two cubs. Or, create your own scary experience in your imagination.

Be mindful of which muscles you activate and what part of your body you are stressing. Then, even all of that out. I suspect you will discover that your mobility will be enhanced significantly as some symptoms show a welcome resolution.

Have fun as you continue to notice the balance between your right and the left sides and as you continue admiring and appreciating your feet.

Center of Gravity

The mindfulness challenge this week is to become more aware of your center. By this I mean your center of gravity. This particular mindfulness practice will yield immeasurable returns if you are currently struggling with balance or mobility problems. No medicines are required. No visits to healthcare practitioners are necessary. The treatment is free and offers benefits which are immediate.

This is an exercise for everyone even if you are not currently experiencing mobility challenges. Athletic superstars are intimately connected with the center of their gravity. Ballerinas, performers and all other individuals who have to be physical in all respects know where their center of their gravity is located.

I suspect you are well aware that the center of gravity is not at the tip of your little finger or the tip of your little toe. It is certainly not at the extremities of your body and it is certainly not in our head (which is where many of us prefer to hang out all the time).

The center of gravity actually resides for most people a couple of inches below their belly button. This place has a name called the tan tien. It is a point in the body that does not have an affiliation or an identity with any specific

22

organ like a heart or a lung; it is an energetic place in everyone's physical body.

Martial artists are very familiar with this place known as the tan tien. It is the source of their power. I suspect many of you have seen martial artists throwing a person from one corner of a room to the other by the flip of their finger. How do they do that? They don't do it by the strength of their finger. They accomplish such an amazing feat by marshaling a power that resides from this place of the tan tien. It is the source of martial art magic.

Using your intention locate your tan tien two inches below your belly button. It is in the middle of your body between the front and the back. Now, fire up your tan tien with the color red - as red as it can possibly become. Fire it up.

- *Feel the red.*
- *Experience the heat.*
- *Connect with the center of your power.*

Become aware of its presence and its existence. When your tan tien is fired up with the frequency that is equivalent to the color red you become centered. You are balanced. It will be quite challenging to fall or to freeze or to confront any mobility challenges whatsoever.

Become more aware this week of the center of your gravity which resides in your tan tien two inches below your belly button in the middle of your body.

- *Know it.*
- *Feel it.*
- *Sense it.*
- *See it*
- *Experience it.*

This same mindfulness practice works for super athletes. You also can access the limitless power that resides in that energetic spot of your body known as the tan tien. Become familiar with your tan tien and you will see miracles happen for yourself this week. Challenge yourself to derive instantaneous benefits. Celebrate the ability to move effortlessly as you fly across the stage of life just like a star ballerina.

You may be thinking - there is no way this can be true. Accept the invitation so you can witness the result. You do not have to confess to anyone that you were wrong! Instead, celebrate the benefits that this mindfulness practice offers.

Implications of Aligning with Your Center of Gravity

When we are not anchored to the center of our gravity, falls, freezing and walking difficulties can very easily emerge. The first deeper meaning of becoming aware of your tan tien and thus becoming anchored to the center of your gravity is that it is much less likely that mobility challenges will be confronted or that falls will be experienced. That is the practical implication of moving the center of your balance to the true center.

The center of gravity is hanging out at the extremities of your body when mobility challenges are confronted. There is no way in the world that you will be able to feel a sense of stability when that happens to be the case. If you currently confront mobility challenges and have an episode that is challenging, the invitation I have for you especially this week and perhaps thereafter is to immediately focus your attention on your tan tien. Shift your center of balance from the extremities to the center of your gravity at your tan tien to attain balance and stability.

There is a second important and profound underlying meaning of becoming sensitive, aware and attentive to your tan tien (which again is two inches below your belly button in the middle of your body). When focused on your tan tien, you cannot be in your head. You cannot be

25

thinking. Rather, you are experiencing the feeling of being centered and grounded.

If you are like me, you have spent most (if not all) of your life in your head thinking about the future, pondering over the past, questioning past actions and solving problems with thoughts that cycle over and over and over again. For people like me, and perhaps like you, this means that the center of our gravity shifts up. In other words, we become top-heavy. Our energy field looks like an inverted pyramid. Is there any wonder this creates mobility challenges?

We also tend to shift the top part of our body back and forth. We become literally twisted from thinking about one thought and one problem to the second thought and second problem - attempting to solve the second problem while continuing to juggle the first thought in our heads. Then of course, the third thought and the fourth problem sneaks in our thoughts to clutter up our life and make us crazy inside.

The twisting eventually becomes problematic. It also takes us away from the present. When mobility challenges emerge, there are fears about something that might happen in the future – for example, a freezing episode or perhaps a fall. That means we are not living in the present moment. We are anticipating the future. This distance from the present makes mobility challenges even more problematic.

26

To remain mindful of the present is the solution. To be attentive to the center of your gravity which resides in your tan tien is the key to maintaining stability whenever you walk, talk, chew or swallow.

Focusing attention on the tan tien (as martial artists do) takes us out of our head. We are usually either commiserating over the past or anticipating the future. It is very rare that we are actually centered in the present moment.

I often see double if not triple rainbows that are seen across the back yard where we have a view of the Puget Sound. These are spectacular images that I have never seen before in my life. When they emerge, the key for me is to be present to the grandeur and the gloriousness of the image of all the colors that emerge in the first, then the second, then third rainbow.

But, when I say out loud,

> *"My, isn't that a pretty rainbow?"*

I am suddenly taking myself out of the present moment. Focusing attention on my tan tien is a way to maintain mindfulness of being present—now. When I am present to the moment, stress cannot rear its ugly head.

Continue then to fire up that tan tien in your body. Strengthen your martial arts power. When we move down

27

from the continuous rattletrap of thoughts that juggle around in our mind second by second and shift attention to the center of our body, we feel secure. We feel safe. We are safe.

By the way, we also become imminently more creative because we are not so scattered and unfocused. Try it. I'm quite sure you will like it. And let me also remind you, no medicine is required. No investment necessary. No travel to a health care provider is needed. This is something you can do for yourself anytime, anywhere.

Space

The mindfulness challenge this week has far reaching implications. My challenge for this week is to become more aware of space. We typically focus our attention on objects, on their physicality. For example, if we are sitting at a table, we are focused on the physical aspects and character of the table and all of the surroundings: the chairs around the table, the objects on the table, trinkets that may have been placed on top of other tables that are nearby. In other words, when we look, we see the physical objects that occupy the space that engulfs us, not the space itself.

Switch that habit. Switch your channel of attention this week. Focus instead on the space around the objects. One of the ways to do this exercise (and to discover the power of its hidden implications) is to focus on the leaves or the branches of a tree. We typically look at the branches or leaves. As you look at trees this week, redirect the focus of your attention to the spaces between the leaves or the branches. You will have to stand still for a few minutes to pull off this observational task.

Look at the space that surrounds objects and you will be amazed at how your consciousness shifts. Be aware of space everywhere as you go through your week, day in and day out.

29

May you have a delightful and exciting time becoming more aware of the many wonders of the world. There are millions more wonders than seven!

Deeper Meaning Behind Space

What is the deeper meaning behind the mindfulness challenge this week of paying attention to the space that surrounds objects? The implications of this exercise are actually profound.

We spend our lives focusing our attention on the physical objects that we see in front of our eyes. We believe that is all there is. Our perceptions guide us to believe that what we think to be physical is solid. We misinterpret the reality of that physical object. We unconsciously believe that it is packed with molecules that are nested together, side by side.

The reality is that any physical object is actually composed of far, far, far more space than the physical aspects of its configuration. I am even here talking about solid objects such as steel and rocks that we typically think are compacted physically. They are not.

This is also true of our bodies. We think of our bodies as pretty solid in their configuration and constitution. The reality is there is far, far, far more space in our bodies than matter in the form of tissues and cells that take on a physical form.

30

When we look at our physical world we believe that anything which exists takes on a solid, physical form. We believe that our bodies are solid when in fact, the space that occupies our bodies constitutes far, far, far, far more of what we are than the physical aspect of our being.

We tend to get attached to certain objects and possessions. For example, many of us have animals. We get attached to those animals. We feel as though that is largely what constitutes joy in our life – our animals, the love and compassion that they return to us that is unqualified. And yet, the reality is that even within the space of those animals there is a significant universe we never see or acknowledge.

When we begin to observe space, then, we open up our awareness to the reality that there is an existence far beyond the reality of our own limited perceptions. This is particularly important when it comes to thought forms. You see, we tend to attach ourselves to specific thoughts,

- *"I'm not good enough."*
- *"I haven't accomplished enough."*
- *"People don't appreciate who I am or what I am."*
- *"I'm really not able to manifest what it is that I have always dreamed of manifesting."*
- *"I wanted to be a piano player. I can never do that now because my fingers are too rigid."*
- *"I wanted to be a singer but I can't do that now because my voice is horse and soft"*

31

- *Et cetera. Et cetera.*

These thoughts all limit us. We do this to ourselves.

Think of the space beyond that. Think of the thoughts that are potential thoughts beyond those limiting thoughts. It really opens up endless possibilities and hope for the future. The space, the universe, the realities out there that we are unaware of - are limitless.

This is a new time for everyone. This is a time in the universe and in the world that is unprecedented. We are seeing change in the world that is miraculous.

Be open to the space that you have not acknowledged heretofore. Watch all of your stress dissolve over what you cannot accomplish minute by minute, day by day, week by week. Stress cannot exist when we hold the reality in our consciousness that endless possibilities exist.

Hand Watching

Hand watching can indeed be a fascinating pastime and hobby. It is also a much underappreciated gateway into being more mindful. To what extent are you aware of how you talk with your hands? Do you use just the right hand or just the left hand, or like most people, do you talk with both hands? If you are a news broadcaster you have been taught to glue your hands to the desk and not talk with them. Most people however talk with their hands.

Be mindful this week of the extent to which you use your hands when you talk. Watch your hands as you talk. Watch them as they communicate with one another. Notice whether or not you tend to use one hand more than another. If so when?

It is well known in that in Western cultures the male energy tends to be on the right side of the body and female on the left. This seems to be reversed in Eastern cultures. Which hand is your dominant hand when you talk?

When you want to make an important point, which hand do you use to point a finger? Is it the right hand? Or, is it the left hand? Or, do you point with fingers on both hands?

Watch your hands

Notice what they say

Don't just watch your own hands. Watch the hands of other people as they talk. Look at their hands as they have this most intricate dance with one another or as they dance by themselves.

You are probably not paying much attention to your hands when you talk. Much of how we communicate with one another becomes very habitual. You will probably discover ways that you communicate that were previously unknown to you when you become more mindful of how you use your hands when you express yourself. You will likely also gain a deeper appreciation for the richness of information that is conveyed through your hands when you talk.

Enjoy being mindful of your hands this week as you are present to each and every month. Allow stress to vanish and dissolve.

Deeper Meaning Behind Hand Watching

What have been your observations from this mindfulness exercise this week which invited you to be more observant of your hands while you talk and the hands of others when they talk? Here's my observation. If you'd asked me before I invented this exercise,

"To what extent do I use my hands when I talk?"

I probably would have reported I don't use them very much. I prefer to use my big mouth.

The truth is, as I observe myself, that I use my hands a great deal when I talk. I'm not even aware of the extent to which my hands facilitate my ability to communicate meaning to others. Has that been your realization too?

Perhaps you have not learned a lot about how you communicate as much as how others communicate. Perhaps you now know much more about how somebody who is particularly close to you expresses themselves through their hands? Perhaps you never realized how much that individual uses their hands to express their feelings and their thoughts?

Our bodies are just like our hands when we talk. The reality is our body is always functioning without our awareness. We do not need to turn on or off any switches for our body to keep on functioning. We do not need to consciously coordinate the pumping of the heart or the exhalation of our breath, or the circulation of our blood. Think of what a monstrous task that would be. It would surely require the participation and the input of an entire population of a very large country to control the physical function of just one human body.

The body is a miracle and yes, we are not aware of everything that it actually does nor do we need to be. Our body knows how to heal itself. All we have to do is to honor that incredible ability. The right side communicates with the left side. The top (head) communicates with the bottom (feet). The body is always in a continuous state of adjustment, always striving to maintain that golden place of balance.

Yes, sometimes our body does need to have some help from us. It is possible that there are so many toxins, bacteria and trauma trapped in our body that it is unable to function. The load is simply too much for the body to handle. Traumatic experiences may be trapped within the cells of the body. If our body is continuously frightened and frozen in a state of perpetual fear, chances of maintaining balance and harmony are slim. The presence of bacteria, fungus and viruses can also interrupt and obstruct the ability of the body to function.

Know in your heart, soul and mind that the body really does have a superior intelligence that far surpasses our own! We can never be aware of precisely what it doing or how it does it. You see, it is all a miracle.

Most of your body, my body and everyone's body who is alive today is actually working perfectly right now. There are some functions that may not be quite in order. Yes, there is work to be done in the form of therapies, in the form of coming back into balance and centeredness, in the

36

form of doing regular meditations, in the form of reducing stress. All of that is important and it is certainly important to discharge, release, remove and eject all negative thoughts that are not in our best and highest good.

Yes it is possible to come back into that golden place of perfect harmony, balance and wellness. This then turns out to be the deeper meaning of the exercise this week to notice your hands. They do what they do and we're not even aware of it. How magical is that?

Have a magnificent time the rest of the week as you even more closely and meticulously watch what your hands do from moment to moment. Watch others as they communicate with their own hands. And most importantly, celebrate the miracle of your body which is working perfectly right now.

Aging

Start with yourself this week as I invite you to track evidence of aging, moment to moment, day to day. When I say start with yourself, the next time that you look at yourself in a mirror ask yourself:

- *How have I been aging recently?*
- *Do I have a wrinkle or two more than I could remember yesterday?*
- *Do I have a gray hair or two more than I can remember just last month?*
- *Are my eyelids droopy?*
- *Is my jaw sagging?*

Look at yourself. Go ahead and be critical if you want. Ask yourself the question,

"How have I been aging?"

Record your observations if you will - whatever observations you would like to make about your own aging. Then, put that record of observations aside.

For the remainder of the week collect evidence of aging that can be found throughout your world. For example,

- Notice paint on walls. Detect evidence of paint that may be fading or chipping.

- Notice dogs. Every dog you pass, ask yourself, *"What's the evidence of aging here? Does this dog have gray hair? Perhaps they are having a problem keeping up with their owner during the walk?"*
- Notice evidence of aging in trees. What evidence is there of aging in trees that you are drawn to observe? Is there moss growing on the branches? Are the branches ragged with age?
- Notice vegetables in your refrigerator. Vegetables spoil when left uneaten.
- Notice expiration dates on products that you purchase at the store. Many food products have expiration dates because food spoils past a certain date.
- Notice neon signs that might have letters missing. After all, the neon signs did not have letters missing when they were new. Now that they have aged it is very common for neon signs to have a flicker in a letter or two or a letter that refuses to light up.
- Notice the petals on flowers which are wilting. Flowers are beautiful but they never last forever.
- Notice the fruit that you eat this week. If left uneaten, fruit eventually rots and discolors.
- Notice cars. Clearly some cars are new; they have just been manufactured. Other cars are decades old and have significant evidence of rust.

Acknowledge all evidence of aging as you go through your daily routine this week, minute by minute, day by day throughout the entire week. Be sure to have fun as you assume the role of a meticulous detective who has a keen eye toward tracking evidence of aging in pretty much everything you encounter.

Deeper Meaning Behind Aging

Did you take my suggestion and look at yourself in the mirror? I did. What did you discover? What were your observations?

I'll tell you what mine were. As I looked, I saw my receding hairline and I zeroed in on my wrinkles. Every time I look in the mirror I worry about that receding hairline. I think to myself the same thought,

> "Oh my goodness, I think it's receding even more this month. I'm not going to have any hair left in just a year or two."

What were your worries? How did you expand and expound upon what you observed to be evidence of aging when you looked at yourself in the mirror?

I have a big secret for you and it goes something like this. If I take what worries me – in my case my receding hairline – and I ask a loved one,

> "So, what do you think about my receding hairline? Doesn't it just drive you crazy?"

What do you suppose they are going to say? I can tell you in an instant. They are going to say,

"Huh? What? What do you mean receding hairline? I like your receding hairline. I think it's distinguished. I don't look at that and think oh my God you're getting older. That's not how I interpret that whatsoever."

Perhaps I'm going to be brazen and I'll then just stretch my point a bit,

"But what about my wrinkles?"

You know what I'm likely to hear? The response is more than likely going to be,

"What wrinkles?"

Perhaps I might want to press even further.

"You know, I've got more and more wrinkles on my forehead."

Very likely the response I'm going to hear is,

"Hmm, I hadn't noticed any wrinkles on your forehead."

You see, others tell us the truth of the meaning that we attribute to aging. We are very adept at creating stress in our life for reasons that do not even exist!

The reality is everything around us including our bodies, is aging. There is simply no way around it. If we zero in at any point in our lives, we can likely recall similar anxieties about our body falling apart.

Go back to the time when you were five years old. Your body was changing then too. You may very likely have had a thought at the age of five of missing something all of a sudden that you liked about your body the month before. We seem to always be judging what it is that we think we see about ourselves. Those judgments almost always have no merit and no meaning to others whatsoever.

Everything around us is aging and changing. It is the way of the world and has always been the way of the world.

1. There is birth.
2. There is life.
3. There is death.

If we continue to live our lives by making assessments of how bad it is that certain trappings of aging are evident, we discredit the beauty of what life is all about.

Better yet, cast all judgments aside for they have no meaning whatsoever to others. Take in the essence of whatever is encountered. Consider looking at yourself again in the mirror - as will I - and ask yourself,

"What's here now? Look at this! What's here now?"

Take in the essence, the beauty and the miracle of what you see.

Aging is something that will always be here for us, for others and for every living entity in the world. Stop fighting it. Take in the full essence of all that is. When you do just that, you will find your life force will explode. Cast out the judgments that block the explosion of your life force.

Let your life force flourish by being present each moment,

- **Accepting**
- **Reveling**
- **Celebrating**
- **Admiring**

All that is in this quite magnificent place that we live called planet earth.

Has your work on these exercises been stress free? Has it been helpful in reducing your symptoms? I certainly hope so! This is the primary reason I developed the mindfulness exercises in the first place.

If you struggled with pacing out these mindfulness exercises so as not to induce more stress, there are several Parkinsons Recovery programs that might help expedite your recovery. My Parkinsons Recovery Mindfulness Program sends the mindfulness exercises in an email to you each and every week. The initial exercise is sent to your email address on day one of the week and the deeper implications are sent four days later. The Parkinsons Recovery Mindfulness Program takes one full year to complete as each exercise is introduced one week at a time. For more information visit:

www.stress.parkinsonsrecovery.com

Parkinsons Recovery Memberships involve a variety of support websites that are essential to recovery. A difference mindfulness exercise is posted each week. For more information on Parkinsons Recovery memberships visit:

www.parkinsonsrecovery.org

Of course, the approach that works for many people is to purchase a single volume of the Parkinsons Recovery

45

Mindfulness program at a time as you have already done! See the introduction for a listing of all nine Parkinsons Recovery Mindfulness volumes.

Thank you for Your Support

On behalf of the thousands of followers of Parkinsons Recovery, I want to thank you for your purchase of this booklet. One hundred percent (100%) of the profits purchases of my books and programs help subsidize the many free services I offer through Parkinsons Recovery -

www.parkinsonsrecovery.com

For information about other products, services and programs visit -

www.parkinsonsrecovery.me

www.ingramcontent.com/pod-product-compliance
Lightning Source LLC
Chambersburg PA
CBHW070232290526
45789CB00004B/1595